THE COMPLETE GUIDE TO GUA SHA:
Ancient Healing Techniques for Health, Beauty, and Vitality

Melanie Wesley

1

Table of Contents

CHAPTER ONE

INTRODUCTION

Gua signifies 'scratch' and Sha implies 'petechiae' (little, level red, purple spots) in Chinese. "Gua Sha started as a full body treatment which an extensive number people don't grasp since facial methods have really become eminent. The central issue is to scratch the skin customarily the upper back to empower circulatory framework, discharge heat-hurts, reinforce lymphatic waste, instigate different indications of the body, and pass solid cells on to the area by invigorating a protected reaction. Occasionally this development makes some staining on the skin, which can look significant. Regardless, have sureness, there is no worsening and the petechiae by and large disappear quickly."

THE BEST SYSTEM TO USE A GUA SHA INSTRUMENT

Right now's not the tremendous chance to blame all power. "I propose clients unbendingly follow the headings of the contraption they have, and to not make up their own system. It is major to go in a vertical, outward bearing just and press warily by drifting over facial oil. Need very heading? work with fragile strain (rather than scratching) and float over the face structures, working inwards and outwards to make a flushing of the skin and swear off making," proposes Vassanelli.

Lying on your front on a wonderful treatment bed, using a most respected scented oil, long strokes with a Gua Sha contraption along your back, arms, legs and neck. Gua Sha ought to be conceivable dependably, in spite of how there are a few sections to consider. "The repeat of Gua Sha truly depends on how enduringly the instrument is used. The more gigantic and more grounded that the strain is of the scratching enhancements applied, the more distinguishable the presence of red etchings which require several days to pick. Along these lines, firm gua sha can be applied a giant number of weeks." Expecting Gua Sha is applied incredibly more mindfully, at standard stretches works brilliantly." You can in like manner use your judgment considering the issue(s) being made due. The authenticity of the issue being stayed aware of may require more ceaseless Gua Sha application. In any case, recall that these tips are for sound skin Gua Sha. "We suggest seeing a supported TCM capable for the utilization of Gua Sha for all clinical related concerns. Adding that it's best wrapped up with another TCM common practice: The best strategy for having Gua Sha for maximal impact and correcting is where it is sought along with needle treatment and performed by an endorsed acupuncturist."

CHAPTER TWO

DOES GUA SHA LEAVE WOUNDS

Gua Sha makes not much of secondary effects, but rather it can wound the skin. "It can on occasion leave wounds since you are squeezing hard, pushing and scratching the skin," sorts out Vassanelli and sees that injuries can be "a pleasant sign that the treatment is working. When done regularly, the readiness can cause ruckuses of exhaustion, due to being overpowered tolerating poisonous substances are conveyed excessively speedy from the body.

WHY IS GUA SHA SO FAMOUS

It could have something to do with the very way by which clear it is. We utilize such a lot of improvement, it's perfect to have a break and utilize a successful, facilitating device that shouldn't stress over to be charged. Also, howdy, those cut outcomes are awesome, as well. "Other than the utilization of Gua Sha in TCM workplaces, we can correspondingly remember this strategy for our managing oneself administrations. Gua Sha is particularly successful at easing major areas of strength for up and separating scarf bonds ideal for those with tight muscles, sluggish dispersing, and tech necks. "As facial treatment, it helps depuff, invigorate microcirculation, and advance collagen creation. The way to Gua Sha is consistency." as such, feel free to get to scraping. The Parts of the "Holographic Meridian Scratching Treatment"

1. Picked nature: Brief preface to the data on viscera, meridians and centers in traditional Chinese prescription, speculation of holographic end and treatment; head discussion of the treatment and clinical idea piece of scratching treatment; systematic prelude to the major perspective for the holographic meridian scratching treatment; picking a titanic social gathering of strong strategies for scratching for wrecks in both Chinese and Western reaction for embody a mix of

unrest division and condition differentiation; and summarizing the clinical idea scratching procedures. It is a reasonable handbook of gua sha.

2. Sharp: Applying the hypotheses of Chinese and Western medicine to figure out the clinical benefits and treatment framework and clinical inspirations driving scratching treatment; introducing totally the sensible controls, things for thought, and signs and contraindications of the scratching treatment. Here are introduced representative wrecks in different clinical divisions, for which scraping treatment has a typical fixing influence and the solid frameworks for scratching for these issues. Stress is placed on disorder differentiation in Western

strategy and issue section in Chinese medicine, which should be participated in clear application. In spite of how there are more than 140,000 difficult situations known to modem approach, all problems are related with brokenness of the 14 meridians and inside organs, according to standard Chinese medication icine. The object of scratching treatment is to address the disharmony in the meridians and inside organs to recover the in general regular gigantic functions. Consequently, the scratching of a lot of meridian centers can be used to treat various contaminations. In the part on clinical application some spot near 100 kinds of customary torments are discussed, but the asserted number is by and large more than that.

3. Reliable: Using clear language and a great deal of pictures and plans to guarantee that perusers can emphatically leam, recall and apply the standards of scratching treatment. In any case far reaching they master the methodologies figured out in Region Three, perusers with close to no clinical data can apply scratching treatment to themselves or others, concerning the photographs in Parts Four and Five. Other than scratching treatment, typical treatment for every issue or condition is figured out and may be used in mix in with the scratching systems.

To give this clinical idea framework to dependably more people and to similarly stimulate standard Chinese medicine respected they have changed and restored this book in the spirit serious areas of strength for of. They perceive that they could zero in on the clinical benefits of mankind with this standard treatment which has no extemporaneous effects and causes no contamination.

STANDARD CHINESE PRESCRIPTION ELECTIVE ARRANGEMENT OR OLD GETTING IT

Qi and Meridians

Qi (conferred and a huge piece of the time made as chi) suggests the fundamental force of the body. It's as a rule mis-fathomed to suggest "soul" or "soul" when it reality, more like an outrageous blood goes through the body. It goes through the body along the meridian lines, as well as through various channels. The nuances of qi alone can be a lifetime study, and it's extremely far past the level. All you genuinely need to know is this: qii s energy that progressions through the body and it are frantic to Chinese medicine. So What Kinds of Meds Could I at whatever point eventually expect from Chinese Cure? As a thorough treatment, Standard Chinese Blueprint works with a puzzling part of cures. Coming up next is a couple:

Neighborhood drug this consolidates the utilization of flavors, roots, mushrooms and other standard things for their strong worth. Several extraordinary animal parts and minerals may as such be used, some of which are particularly hazardous. There are normal solutions for treat all around affliction and condition known to clinical science, and, vastly, some that aren't.

Needle treatment this is the exhibit of presenting needles especially little ones into express obsessions along the body. Normal needle treatment follows the meridian lines indicated quite a bit early, yet present day experts are adding their own opportunity to their method. Needle treatment is typically used for steady wretchedness, mental issues, or other material improvement issues. Its redder hot embellishments will propose it for by and large whatever else, as well. Investigating is a curious sort of back rub/detoxification. This requires splendid glass cups which have the air inside warmed by a fire or smoke. While warm inside, they are placed on the back where they then, suck up the skin into the cup. A piece of the more present day office correspondingly use cups with siphons presented. Expected to clean the scope of harmful substances, it's not upheld enduring you need to go to the sea side: it leaves tremendous enormous red circles regularly down your back!

Gua sha-Another astonishing treatment, gua sha is the most prominent system for directing scouring the skin with smooth bits of jade, stone, bone or tusk. Its start and end except for a fragile treatment, reliably achieving chafing making or red etchings on the skin. Its evident useful use is amazingly wide, finally, as it is be used for all that from irritating environment to cholera. Not a treatment for those with a low upsetting impact edge!

Physical and Breathing exercises - Standard Chinese Medicine other than stays mindful of its pre-arranged specialists/patients to take part in sound turn of events. For the stream and concordance of qi, notwithstanding, the ideal exercises will do. Taichi, qigong, yoga, appraisal and hand to hand drawing in are very seen as shocking exercises inside Standard Chinese Blueprint, as is reflection and different breathing exercises.

IS STANDARD CHINESE APPROACH SAFE

Standard Chinese Fix is... strategy. That truly expects that at whatever point used unequivocally, it can have striking consistent worth. In any case, like any medicine used mistakenly, it will by and large be risky. Continually counsel clinical idea specialists going prior to starting any new treatment.

Standard Chinese Fix has the extra bet of being less coordinated. Tricks and washouts succeed, so it's as essential to check insistences as watchfully as a couple of other clinical benefits capable you see. Fundamentally, this lack of pick suggests that different Chinese clinical practices are in ordinary untested by standard analysts. This suggests that the arrangements can go from essential, to unimportant, or even to noxious. Again thought and sharp inspiration should be your associate.

IS STANDARD CHINESE REACTION FOR ME

Put forward surely: maybe. Between drug audits, ace mix-ups, and taking off clinical costs, different people are going to elective fixes. They can help a patient in various ways. For unequivocal people, regardless, it may not be the best choice. For those with infuriating conditions, for instance, compromising development or silly conditions like a broke reference fragment, Western fix truly has an unmatched history. In any case, it doesn't mean these fixes can't be animated with Traditional Chinese Answer for as a rule unmistakable effect. Finally, the choice genuinely relies upon you and your clinical benefits plan.

CHAPTER THREE

GRASTON METHOD HELPS IN RELIEF FROM DISCOMFORT

At the point when an individual is harmed, the body sets down stringy scar tissue to safeguard the injury. Scar tissue grips can happen from microtrauma, as redundant movement wounds, for example, swimming, tennis or golf swings, or from macrotrauma, for example, a torn muscle or gruff injury from falling or in physical games like football and lacrosse. The scar tissue restricts the scope of movement, and in many occasions causes torment, which keeps the patient from working as the person did before the injury.

At the point when seen under a magnifying lens, ligaments and tendons have thick, extended filaments running in a similar course. At the point when the delicate tissue is harmed, it can recuperate in an erratic example, bringing about limited scope of movement, scarring and torment. The scar tissue makes sense of why numerous wounds feel "unique" even after weeks or long periods of obvious mending.

Another delicate tissue treatment called The Graston Procedure integrates the old Chinese treatment of Gua Sha, cross-erosion back rub, and current innovation into a delicate tissue treatment that has been standing out. The treated steel Graston Strategy instruments have been used by in excess of 50 significant expert and novice sports associations. Coaches, actual specialist, alignment specialists and clinicians at these associations are treating first class competitors consistently and relying on the Graston Procedure to get them injury free, permitting them to contend at the best presentation levels.

The Graston Method's instruments are utilized to improve the clinician's capacity to recognize scar tissue, grips and delicate tissue limitations in the impacted regions. Gifted bone and joint specialists and advisors utilize the hardened steel instruments to bald spot and "catch" fibrotic tissue, which promptly distinguishes the areas of limitation. When the tissue has been distinguished, the instruments are utilized to separate the fibrotic scar tissue with the goal that it tends to be consumed by the body. Patients normally get 2-3 medicines each week north of 4-5 weeks; be that as it may, most patients have a positive reaction by the third or fourth treatment.

WHERE TO FIND REMARKABLE BACK RUB ADMINISTRATIONS

On the off chance that you have a muscle protest, you'll most likely have thought about rub as your most memorable port of call. Individuals all around the world visit masseuses consistently to keep their body moving, whether they wind up afflicted by pressure cerebral pains, sports wounds, or they're attempting to financially recover after a mishap - this old treatment can work supernatural occurrences. Be that as it may, in the event that not executed accurately, the outcomes can frustrate. Frequently the primary spot somebody will go for this extravagance is a lodging or spa. And keeping in mind that these normal medicines are brilliant for assisting you with unwinding, they are not generally embraced by those with top to bottom information on the life systems, so the impacts don't will more often than not stand the test of time. While usually rehearsed medicines, like Swedish back rub, are viable at treating shallow muscle protests, procedures like Profound Tissue medicines will venture through them and into the hidden muscles underneath, which could be the wellspring of your aggravation. This sort of treatment requires progressed ability and information, so isn't presented by all specialists.

On the off chance that you endure with a longstanding issue, or are in torment excessively intense to try and consider allowing somebody to apply strain to your distressed region, you ought to focus on an expert in kinesiology to assist with restoring you of your uneasiness. There are a scope of various ways to deal with knead not simply Profound Tissue or Swedish back rub and some of the time it takes a specialist to view as the right one.

Finding an autonomous, enlisted practitioner is ideal. These can frequently be searched out secretly, yet are definitely worth the speculation. Furthermore, these practices are by and large run by experts who are intrigued for the most part in lessening your aggravation. Furthermore, in spite of the fact that they also will have bills and a home loan to pay, they are more worried about treating the issue than charging you for bunches of additional items. Attempt to find a specialist who will charge you a level expense for the meeting length, for example an hour, and who will toss in a free counsel. You might find that your advisor needs to counsel your particular issue toward the start of every meeting. This isn't on the grounds that they're being lethargic or that they have failed to remember what the issue it, it's so they can treat every meeting freely of the last, surveying your aggravation level and resilience on that specific day. The most all around rehearsed advisors will comprehend that your aggravation will change from one day to another. Frequently possibly 14 days might slip by among meetings, and your concern might have deteriorated during that time. So in spite of the fact that you might find it disappointing to rehash the same thing, you will before long begin to see the advantages of moving toward every meeting as an independent treatment. Professionals will frequently be knowledgeable, in kinesiology, yet in addition in physiology and muscular as well. They will probably have an abundance of involvement working with bone and joint specialist and specialists to help those restoring from wounds and tasks. This experience will give them an unmistakable edge against traditional specialists, who will more often than not offer just a single type of treatment. Specialists in motor back rub will actually want to give various medicines, and will work with you to conclude which is appropriate for you.

Procedures might incorporate Games Back rub, Trigger Point Treatment, Profound Tissue or Gua Sha a customary Chinese clinical treatment exceptionally viable at easing torment. Be that as it may, the best medicines will be custom fitted to your body's particular necessities, and will not follow a particular daily schedule. This is one more advantage to searching out a confidential masseuse, as they won't treat any two bodies something similar. Experts in this area will grasp the requirement for a remarkable treatment, and will actually want to give knowledge into what your body needs to keep up its solidarity.

THE END

www.ingramcontent.com/pod-product-compliance
Lightning Source LLC
Chambersburg PA
CBHW070755260726
48660CB00007B/3135